10-Minutes Wall Pilates Workout for Seniors

Discover Gentle and Effective Pilates Exercises Tailored for Seniors and Improve Your Well-being in Just 10 Minutes a Day with Wall-Based Workouts

Jerry Hargrave

Disclaimer:

The information provided in this book, although fully accurate , is for informational purposes only. It is not intended to be a substitute for professional medical advice, diagnosis, or treatment. Always seek the advice of your physician or other qualified health provider with any questions you may have regarding a medical condition. Never disregard professional medical advice or delay in seeking it because of something you have read in this book.

The publisher and author are not responsible for any injuries or damages arising from the use of the information contained in this book. Readers assume full responsibility for their own health and well-being.

THIS BOOK BELONGS TO

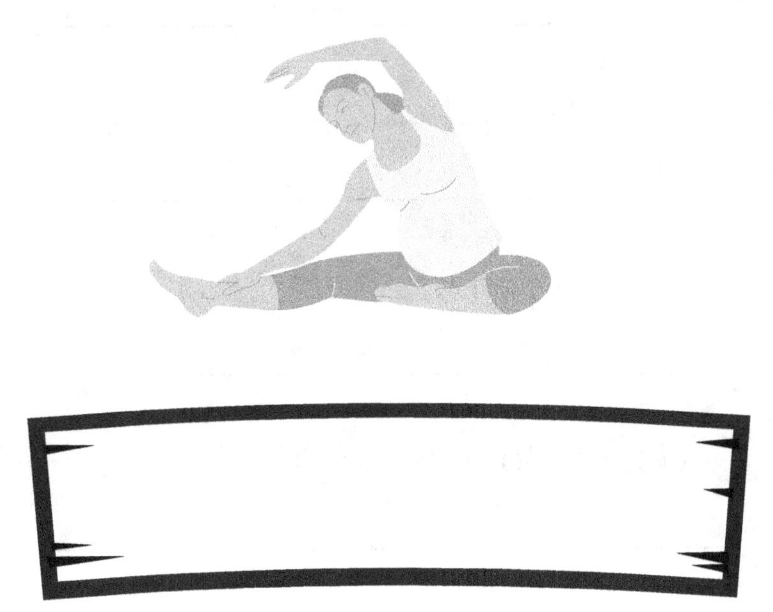

Table of Contents

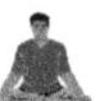

Introduction

Hello, Welcome to Wall Pilates for Seniors in 10 Minutes! I am Jerry Hargrave and it is my pleasure to assist you through this route towards improved fitness as well as health. But before we start let me quickly tell you a little bit about myself and how pilates has completely transformed my life.

A few years ago, at the beginning of my fifties I noticed that I was starting to experience typical age related problems i.e. stiffness, decreased mobility and nagging aches and pains. Thus like many people my age, I wanted a way of staying healthy but not going overboard. That's when I discovered Pilates; it changed everything. Pilates is more than just exercising; it is an overall approach to wellness that stresses on core strength, flexibility and body awareness. It's mild yet highly effective thus very suitable for individuals of our age.

My personal journey with Pilates soon turned into a love affair with the exercise which led me into becoming a certified instructor. Essentially I hoped to enlighten people in their geriatric years about the advantages associated with practicing Pilates which include enhanced strength, posture alignment as well as increased energy levels. There were some astonishing differences in my clients over time. Because of freedom of movement offered by pilates they have seen themselves regain self-esteem, confidence, improve their standing balance and even discover new interests.

In this book, I've compiled a collection of 10-minute Wall Pilates workouts tailored specifically for seniors.

These workouts are gentle but effective, focusing on improving balance, flexibility, and strength without putting too much strain on the joints. This collection is suitable for both experts and beginners

Each workout is broken down into simple, easy-to-follow exercises that you can do at home with little to no equipment. Whether you only have 10 minutes or an hour, you can easily incorporate these workouts into your daily routine and begin reaping the benefits of Pilates immediately.

But, before we get started with the workouts, I'd like to share a story that shows Pilates' transformative power for seniors. This story is based on one of my experiences as a Pilates instructor.

The Story of Margaret: A Pilates Success Story

Margaret was 68 years old when she first entered my Pilates studio. She was hesitant and unsure, having never done Pilates before. She had been suffering from back pain and a general sense of stiffness, making it difficult for her to enjoy her favorite activities such as gardening and walking in the park.

Margaret was amazed at how quickly her body improved as she began her Pilates journey. Gentle movements and focused breathing helped to relieve muscle tension, and core-strengthening exercises improved her posture and balance.

Margaret's back pain began to subside after just a few weeks of regular Pilates practice, and she felt more free and confident in her movements. Her posture improved, and she felt stronger and more energized than she had in many years.

Margaret's mindset, however, may have been the most significant change. Pilates had changed not only her body, but also her perspective on life. She felt more empowered and in control of her health, and she began to view her age as an opportunity to live life to the fullest.

Margaret is now 78 years old and continues to practice Pilates on a regular basis. She no longer sees her age as an impediment to staying active and healthy, but rather as a blessing that allows her to continue doing the things she enjoys with confidence and energy.

Margaret's story is just one of many that show how Pilates can transform the lives of seniors. Whether you want to improve your strength, flexibility, or overall well-being, Pilates can help you achieve your goals and live your best life.

I invite you to join me on this journey to improved health and vitality. Together, we can realize Pilates' incredible potential and embrace the joy of movement at any age. Let's get started.

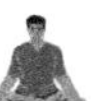

CHAPTER 1: INTRODUCTION TO WALL PILATES

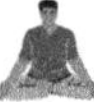

Welcome to the world of Wall Pilates, a gentle yet powerful exercise method designed exclusively for seniors to improve strength, flexibility, balance, and overall well-being. In this detailed introduction, we will look at the core principles of Pilates and how using a wall in your practice may improve stability, support, and safety.

Pilates, created in the early twentieth century, has become well-known for its capacity to strengthen the body's core muscles, improve posture, and increase mind-body awareness. Pilates distinguishes itself by emphasizing precision, control, breath, and flowing movement—all of which contribute to a well-rounded training approach.

As we age, it becomes increasingly vital to focus on workouts that promote joint health, muscle strength, and balance in order to avoid falls and maintain independence. Pilates excels in this regard, providing a low-impact yet highly effective type of exercise that can be tailored to individuals of all fitness levels and abilities.

The use of a wall in Pilates is an excellent tool for seniors, offering extra support, stability, and feedback during exercises. Whether you're new to Pilates or have been training for years, including the wall into your routine will help you deepen your practice and achieve new levels of strength and flexibility.

This chapter will address the following topics:

Let's start by looking at the numerous benefits that Pilates provides to seniors, laying the groundwork for a transforming path to better health and energy.

1.1 Benefits of Pilates for Seniors

Pilates is a comprehensive kind of exercise that benefits not only the physical body but also the mind and spirit. Regular Pilates exercise for seniors can offer numerous benefits that help to general well-being:

Improved Core Strength: The core muscles, which include the abdominals, back, and pelvic floor, are essential for maintaining stability, balance, and posture. Pilates focuses on strengthening these muscles, which can help elders avoid falls and retain independence in daily activities.

Enhanced Flexibility: As we age, our muscles tighten and become less flexible, causing stiffness and discomfort. Pilates uses dynamic stretching motions to extend and elongate the muscles, increasing flexibility and range of movement.

Better Posture: Poor posture is a prevalent problem among seniors, and it can lead to back discomfort, joint stiffness, and reduced mobility. Pilates focuses on optimal alignment and body awareness, which helps to address postural abnormalities and create a more upright and aligned posture.

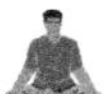

Increased Balance and Stability: As people age, their balance declines, increasing the risk of falls and accidents. Pilates movements require balance and proprioception, which improves stability and reduces the risk of falling.

Joint Health and Mobility: Pilates exercises are easy on the joints while still offering a rigorous workout. Pilates, by lubricating the joints and boosting circulation, can help relieve stiffness and discomfort caused by arthritis and other age-related disorders.

Pilates fosters attentive movement and focused breathing, which promotes relaxation and stress reduction. Pilates provides a vital opportunity for seniors to unwind and refresh both body and mind, especially if they are experiencing increased stress due to health issues or lifestyle changes.

1.2 Understanding the Function of the Wall

Traditional Pilates movements are usually done on a mat or with specific equipment like the Reformer or Cadillac. While each of these tools has its own set of benefits, the wall is a versatile and easily accessible prop that can be utilized to improve the effectiveness of Pilates exercises, especially for seniors.

The wall provides stability and support, allowing seniors to safely perform a variety of activities while maintaining perfect alignment and control. Whether you're working on core strength, balance, or flexibility, the wall may help you feel stable and confident in your exercise.

Furthermore, the wall is an effective tool for proprioceptive feedback, assisting seniors in developing a better understanding of their body's position in space. Using the wall as a reference point allows you to improve your alignment, deepen your stretches, and engage the right muscles more efficiently.

Throughout this tutorial, we will look at many ways to use the wall into your Pilates practice, such as using it for support during standing exercises or for resistance and feedback in seated and supine positions. By embracing the wall as a Pilates partner, you can achieve new levels of strength, stability, and vibrancy.

1.3 Safety Concerns and Precautions

Before starting any new workout routine, especially as a senior, emphasize safety and pay attention to your body's cues. While Pilates is generally regarded safe for most people, certain precautions must be taken to reduce the chance of injury:

contact with Your Healthcare Provider: Before beginning any new workout program, especially if you have pre-existing health ailments or concerns, you should contact with your healthcare provider or a certified fitness professional. They may offer tailored assistance and guarantee that Pilates is fit for your specific needs.

Start Slowly and Progress Gradually: If you're new to Pilates or returning to exercise after a long break, it's ideal to begin slowly and gradually increase the intensity and duration of your exercises. Listen to your body and avoid pushing too hard, especially in the beginning.

Focus on Proper Technique: In Pilates, proper technique is vital for maximizing performance and reducing the danger of injury. Pay close attention to alignment cues and movement instructions, and ask for clarification if necessary. The quality of movement is more essential than quantity.

Modify as needed: Not all exercises will be appropriate for everyone, particularly those who have unique physical restrictions or injuries. Be prepared to alter exercises to meet your body's specific demands and abilities. A trained instructor can assist you in identifying relevant adjustments.

Stay Hydrated and Take Breaks: It's critical to stay hydrated while exercising, especially for seniors who are more prone to dehydration. Take regular water breaks and pay attention to your body's indications for rest and recovery.

By adhering to these safety precautions and taking a careful attitude to your Pilates practice, you can reduce your chance of injury while still reaping the advantages of Pilates well into your senior years.

1.4 Set Up Your Space for Wall Pilates

Creating a designated place for your Pilates practice can assist to set the tone for success and make it simpler to include exercise into your daily routine. While Pilates does not require much equipment or space, there are a few important factors to consider while setting up your room:

Choose a Quiet, Clutter-Free Area: Choose a calm, clutter-free space of your home where you may move freely without interruption. Ideally, you should have enough room to lie down on a mat, arms and legs completely stretched in all directions.

Gather your equipment. Wall Pilates requires minimum equipment, basically a stable wall and sometimes a yoga mat or gym mat for increased comfort. Make sure your wall is free of any obstructions or risks that could impede your actions.

Consider Lighting and Ventilation: Natural light and proper ventilation can help your Pilates practice by creating a pleasant and energizing environment. If feasible, choose a room with plenty of natural light, or use extra lighting as needed. Make sure the room is well-ventilated so you can stay comfortable during your workout.

Establish a Relaxing Ambiance: Set the tone for your Pilates session by integrating elements that promote relaxation and attention. Consider playing relaxing music, burning scented candles, or displaying inspirational quotations or photos that speak to you.

Personalize Your Space: Your Pilates practice area should represent your individual interests and requirements. Add any additional props or accessories that will benefit your practice, such as foam rollers, resistance bands, or Pilates balls. Make it a place where you can feel relaxed, inspired, and driven to move your body.

By devoting time to creating a dedicated Pilates room in your house, you can create an atmosphere that supports your practice and makes it simpler to include exercise into your everyday routine.

1.5 Getting Started: Advice for Beginners

Starting a new workout regimen, whether you're new to Pilates or returning from a hiatus, can be intimidating. However, with the appropriate mindset and approach, you may position yourself for success while enjoying the road to better health and energy. Here are some suggestions to help you get started with your Wall Pilates practice:

Start with the basics: Begin your Pilates adventure by understanding the fundamental movements and principles. Before moving on to more complex exercises, make sure you understand good alignment, breathing techniques, and core engagement.

Take it Slow: Pilates is not about speeding through movements or pushing yourself to exhaustion. Instead, concentrate on moving deliberately and with control, emphasizing the quality of each movement rather than the number. Take breaks as needed and adhere to your body's cues.

Be patient and persistent: Pilates, like any other kind of exercise, requires time and effort to master. Be patient with yourself and acknowledge your minor triumphs along the way. Consistency is crucial, so add Pilates into your regimen on a regular basis, even if it's only for a few minutes per day.

Listen to Your Body: Your body knows best, so follow its cues and modify your practice accordingly. If anything doesn't feel right or causes discomfort, ease up and attempt a modified version of the exercise. Respect your body's boundaries and don't push yourself too hard.

Seek coaching and Support: If you're concerned about proper technique or require individualized coaching, try working with a competent Pilates instructor, either in person or via virtual courses. They can offer useful criticism, suggestions, and encouragement to help you advance safely and productively.

Stay Consistent: Consistency is essential for seeing results in Pilates. Make a commitment to yourself to prioritize your Pilates practice and arrange regular sessions on your calendar. Even on days when you don't feel inspired, getting out and moving your body will help you in the long term.

With these guidelines in mind, you'll be ready to start your Wall Pilates journey with confidence and enthusiasm. Remember that every action you take to improve your health and vitality is a positive one. In the following chapters, we'll look at a range of wall Pilates exercises that will strengthen your body, increase your flexibility, and boost your spirits. Prepare to feel stronger, more balanced, and brighter than ever before!

CHAPTER 2: WARM-UP

Welcome to Chapter 2 of your Wall Pilates journey: the Warm-Up. In this chapter, we'll go over the significance of warming up before exercising, investigate the physiological benefits of a complete warm-up practice, and walk you through a comprehensive sequence of activities meant to prepare your body and mind for the difficulties ahead.

Whether you're new to Pilates or an experienced practitioner, it's critical to prioritize the warm-up phase to ensure that your body is appropriately prepared for the demands of exercise. A well-rounded warm-up serves numerous important functions:

Increase Blood Flow: By gradually boosting your heart rate and circulation, a warm-up helps transport oxygen and nutrients to your muscles, improving performance and efficiency.

Loosen Up Muscles and Joints: During the warm-up phase, gentle motions and dynamic stretches serve to loosen tight muscles and enhance joint mobility, lowering the risk of injury and increasing flexibility.

Activate the Nervous System: Warming up prepares your nervous system for exercise by improving coordination, balance, and proprioception.

Mentally Prepare for Exercise: The warm-up period allows you to focus inward, center your mind, and mentally prepare for the physical obstacles that await you, promoting mindfulness and presence throughout your workout.

2.1 Main Elements Of A Pilates Warm-Up

Cardiovascular Activity: Start your warm-up with 5-10 minutes of light cardiovascular exercise to boost your heart rate and circulation. This could be brisk walking, marching in place, or gentle cycling on a stationary cycle. The idea is to progressively increase your heart rate and warm up your muscles in order to perform more energetic motions.

Dynamic Stretching: After your cardiovascular warm-up, perform a sequence of dynamic stretches that target key muscle groups and joints. Dynamic stretching entails controlled, fluid movements that take your body through its whole range of motion, thereby improving flexibility and mobility. Dynamic stretches include arm circles, leg swings, torso twists, and hip circles.

Joint Mobilization: Include exercises that target the spine, shoulders, hips, and other major joints to improve mobility and range of motion. This could involve modest spinal twists, shoulder rolls, hip circles, and ankle circles. Pay attention to any areas of tightness or restriction, and move with caution to relieve tension and stiffness.

Core Activation: Perform specialized movements to stimulate the deep abdominal muscles, obliques, and pelvic floor. This could include exercises like pelvic tilts, abdominal bracing, and modest core stabilizing motions to activate the muscles that support your spine and pelvis.

Breathing Awareness: Use the warm-up phase to develop breath awareness and establish a rhythmic breathing pattern that will serve you well throughout your Pilates session.

To oxygenate your muscles and induce relaxation, practice deep diaphragmatic breathing, which involves inhaling deeply with the nose and expelling thoroughly through the mouth.

Mindfulness and Centering: At the end of your warm-up, take a few moments to center your mind and direct your attention within. If you're comfortable, close your eyes and take a few deep breaths, focusing on your body's feelings and creating an intention for your Pilates exercise. This minute of awareness can help you approach your workout with more presence, attention, and clarity.

2.2 Sample Warm-up Routine

The Pilates warm-up exercise provided below is intended to prepare your body and mind for a Wall Pilates session. Feel free to adjust the exercises as needed based on your fitness level, mobility, and any special needs or limits you may have.

March in Place (2 minutes): Start by moving in place, with your legs raised and your arms swinging naturally. Land softly and engage your core muscles to help maintain your spine.

Arm Circles (1 minute): Stand tall, feet hip-width apart, and extend your arms out to the sides to shoulder height. Circle your arms forward for 30 seconds, then change direction and circle backward for another 30 seconds. Maintain a relaxed shoulder position and an engaged core throughout.

Leg Swings (1 minute per leg): Stand close to a wall or a solid surface for support.

Swing one leg forward and backward in a controlled manner, letting your hip joint open and close. Repeat for one minute, then move to the opposite leg. Maintain good posture and engage your core to ensure stability.

Cat-Cow Stretch (one minute): Get down on your hands and knees on a mat or cushioned surface. Inhale while arching your back and lifting your gaze to the ceiling (Cow Pose), and exhale as you round your spine and tuck your chin to your chest (Cat Pose). Flow easily between these two postures, harmonizing your breath and movement.

Pelvic Tilts (1 Minute): Stay on your hands and knees and tilt your pelvis forward and backward, progressing from a neutral spine to a gentle arch and eventually a small round. This technique mobilizes the lumbar spine and pelvis while activating the deep core muscles.

Standing Spinal Twist (1 minute per side): Stand tall, feet hip-width apart, arms extended out to the sides. Exhale as you twist your torso to the right, placing your left hand on your right leg and stretching your right arm back behind you. Hold for a few breaths before switching sides and repeating on the opposite side.

Diaphragmatic Breathing (1 minute): Take a comfortable seated or standing position with your spine tall and shoulders relaxed. Place one hand on your chest, the other on your abdomen. Inhale deeply with your nose, allowing your abdomen to expand, then exhale fully through your mouth, bringing your navel closer to your spine. Focus on breathing deeply into your diaphragm, allowing it to expand and contract with each breath.

Mindful Centering (1 Minute):

If you feel comfortable, close your eyes and spend a moment to connect with your breath and body. Scan your body from head to toe for any areas of tightness or discomfort, then exhale intentionally to release any tension. Set an aim for your Pilates practice, whether it's to improve strength, flexibility, balance, or awareness, and carry it with you as you start your workout.

Take your time with each exercise, moving carefully and with intention, and observe how your body reacts to the motions. Remember to breathe deeply and be present during your warm-up ritual, enabling yourself to fully immerse in the moment.

CHAPTER 3: STANDING WALL EXERCISES FOR POSTURE

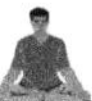

Welcome to Chapter 3 of your Wall Pilates journey, where we'll focus on standing wall exercises that enhance your posture. Good posture is vital for overall health and well-being because it reduces pain and discomfort, promotes good spinal alignment, and boosts confidence and self-esteem. In this chapter, we'll look at a set of ten standing wall exercises that target major muscles involved in maintaining excellent posture, including the core, back, shoulders and hips.

Before we get started with the exercises, let's talk about how important posture is and how these exercises can help you reach and maintain perfect alignment.

Introduction to posture:

Posture is the alignment of your bodily components relative to one another while standing, sitting, or lying down. Maintaining the natural curvature of the spine, evenly distributing your body weight on your feet, and keeping your shoulders relaxed and aligned with your hips are all components of good posture.

Poor posture, on the other hand, can cause a variety of problems, including back discomfort, neck pain, headaches, and limited mobility. Sedentary lifestyles, prolonged sitting, muscle imbalances, and inappropriate alignment all contribute to bad posture over time

The good news is that posture may be improved with targeted workouts and mindful movement methods such as Pilates. Strengthening the muscles that support good alignment and developing body awareness will help you progressively retrain your body to maintain improved posture all day..

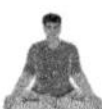

Standing wall exercises are especially useful for improving posture because they use the wall to offer feedback and stability while targeting important muscle groups involved in postural alignment. These exercises assist to strengthen the core, stretch the spine, open the chest, and increase shoulder mobility, resulting in a higher, more upright position.

Now, let's explore 10 standing wall exercises that will help you enhance your posture and feel more confident and balanced in your body.

Wall Squat

10 REPS

Detailed Step by Step Instructions

- Stand with your back to the wall, feet hip-width apart, and arms at your sides.
- Engage your core and carefully slide down the wall into a squat position, bending your knees to 90 degrees.
- Keep your back against the wall and your knees in line with your ankles.
- Hold this position for 15-30 seconds before slowly pushing yourself back to standing.
- Repeat 8-10 times, keeping your weight in your heels and your core engaged throughout.

Notes

Wall Leg Lifts

10 REPS

Detailed Step by Step Instructions

- Stand facing the wall, hands lightly resting against it for support.
- Engage your core and lift one leg straight out in front of you, parallel to the ground.
- Hold this position for a few breaths, then lower your leg to the floor.
- Repeat on the opposite side, alternating legs for 8-10 repetitions per side.
- Maintain a tall spine and steady breathing throughout the movement.

Notes

Wall Calf Raises

10 REPS

Detailed Step by Step Instructions

- Stand facing the wall, hands lightly resting against it for support.
- Lift your heels off the ground and rise up onto the balls of your feet.
- Hold this position for a few breaths, then lower your heels to the floor.
- Repeat 8-10 times, focusing on raising and lowering with control and keeping a strong core throughout.

Notes

Wall Side Leg Lifts

10 REPS

Detailed Step by Step Instructions

- Stand sideways to the wall, one hand resting lightly against it for support.
- Engage your core and raise your upper leg straight out to the side, parallel to the floor.
- Hold this position for a few breaths, then lower your leg to the floor.
- Repeat 8-10 times on each side, focusing on maintaining stability with your supporting leg and keeping your torso erect.

Notes

Wall Side Bend

10 REPS

Detailed Step by Step Instructions

- Stand with your side to the wall, one hand on the wall for support.
- Engage your core and lift the opposite arm above, stretching the side of your body.
- Hold this position for a few breaths until you feel a slight stretch along the side of your torso.
- Return to the beginning posture and continue on the opposite side, switching sides for 8-10 times.
- With each repetition, work on stretching the spine and opening up the side body.

Notes

Wall Hip Flexor Stretch

10 REPS

Detailed Step by Step Instructions

- Stand facing away from the wall, one foot a few feet in front of you and the other pressed against the wall behind you.
- Engage your core and gradually lunge forward with your front leg while keeping your back heel planted on the wall.
- Hold this pose for 15-30 seconds until you feel a stretch in the front of your hips and thighs.
- Repeat on the opposite side, alternating sides for 8-10 times.
- Maintain your torso upright and pelvis level during the stretch.

Notes

Wall Spine Stretch

10 REPS

Detailed Step by Step Instructions

- Stand facing the wall, your feet hip-width apart, and your hands rest lightly against the wall for support.
- Engage your core and slowly circle your spine, lowering your chin into your chest and reaching your tailbone toward the wall.
- Hold this position for a few breaths, feeling the stretch along your spine.
- Return to a neutral spine position, then gradually arch your back, elevating your chest toward the ceiling and bringing your shoulder blades together.
- Hold this pose for a few breaths until you feel a soft opening in your chest and shoulders.
- Repeat the sequence 8-10 times, moving smoothly between rounded and arched postures.

Notes

Wall Shoulder Opener

10 REPS

Detailed Step by Step Instructions

- Stand facing the wall, arms extended aloft and palms pressed onto it.
- Slowly walk your hands along the wall, bringing your chest closer to the wall.
- Hold this pose for a few breaths to feel a deep stretch across your chest and shoulders.
- Return to the beginning posture and repeat 8-10 times, keeping a tall spine and open chest throughout.

Notes

Wall Angel

10 REPS

Detailed Step by Step Instructions

- Stand with your back to the wall, feet hip-width apart, and arms at your sides.
- Press your lower back against the wall and engage your core muscles.
- Slide your arms slowly up the wall, keeping your elbows and wrists in constant touch with the wall.
- Continue to slide your arms overhead, forming a "Y" shape with your biceps adjacent to your ears.
- Hold this stance for a few breaths before slowly lowering your arms back to your sides.
- Repeat 8-10 times, focusing on maintaining contact with the wall and engaging your core throughout.

Notes

Wall Press

10 REPS

Detailed Step by Step Instructions

- Stand facing the wall, feet hip-width apart, arms outstretched in front of you at shoulder height, palms pressed into the wall.
- Engage your core and firmly press your palms into the wall while leaning slightly forward.
- Hold this pose for a few breaths to feel a mild stretch across your chest and shoulders.
- Slowly push yourself away from the wall, returning to your starting position.
- Repeat 8-10 times, focusing on keeping a long spine and a strong core throughout.

Notes

CHAPTER 4: WALL STRETCHES

In today's sedentary lifestyle, many people spend long periods of time sitting at desks or doing activities that can cause muscular tightness and stiffness, especially in the neck, shoulders, and back. Wall stretches are a set of movements that use a wall as support to relieve tension and improve flexibility in certain areas. These stretches are simple to include into your regular routine and are especially good for those who suffer from discomfort caused by extended sitting or repeated movements.

Moreover, incorporating wall stretches into your routine can also promote better posture and alignment by lengthening tight muscles and releasing tension that may be pulling the body out of alignment. By regularly practicing these stretches, you can help counteract the negative effects of prolonged sitting and repetitive movements, leading to improved mobility, reduced discomfort, and a greater sense of well-being in your daily life.

In this chapter, we'll look at ten wall stretches and provide extensive step-by-step directions to ensure good technique and maximum efficiency.

Wall Chest Stretch

30 SECONDS –1 MINUTE

Detailed Step by Step Instructions

- Stand around arm's length from a wall, with your feet hip-width apart for support.
- Place your right palm and forearm on the wall at shoulder height, fingers pointing to the ceiling.
- Gently shift your body away from the wall to the left, keeping your arm against it.
- As you spin, concentrate on expanding your chest and experiencing a stretch over the front of your right shoulder and chest.
- Keep your shoulders relaxed and your spine straight.
- Hold the stretch for 30 seconds to 1 minute, allowing your muscles to slowly relax and extend.
- Remember to breathe deeply and evenly during the stretch.
- After finishing the stretch on one side, switch to the opposite side to maintain bodily symmetry and balance.

Notes

Wall Shoulder Stretch

30 SECONDS –1 MINUTE

Detailed Step by Step Instructions

- Stand sideways to the wall, with your right side facing it.
- Extend your right arm and place your palm flat against the wall at shoulder height.
- Keep your feet grounded and your body stable as you gently rotate away from the wall, using your arm as leverage.
- Feel the stretch across the front of your right shoulder and chest, as well as along the side of your torso.
- Avoid overarching your back or straining your neck; instead, focus on maintaining a neutral spine.
- Hold the stretch for 30 seconds to 1 minute, breathing deeply and allowing the tension to release gradually.
- Switch sides to stretch the left shoulder and chest, ensuring balanced flexibility on both sides of your body.

Notes

Wall Upper Back Stretch

30 SECONDS.

Detailed Step by Step Instructions

- Stand facing the wall, arms outstretched at shoulder height, palms against the wall.
- Take a step back with your feet, keeping your arms straight, and allow your torso to bend forward slightly from the hips.
- Engage your core muscles to keep your spine stable and prevent overarching.
- Feel the stretch in your upper back, between your shoulder blades, and through your shoulders.
- To find the best stretch for your body, try shifting your weight gently from side to side or up and down.
- Hold the pose for 30 seconds to a minute, focusing on relaxing any tension you may be experiencing.
- Maintain consistent breathing during the stretch, inhaling deeply to extend your ribcage and exhaling fully to relieve any tension.

Notes

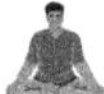

Wall Lat Stretch

30 SECONDS.

Detailed Step by Step Instructions

- Stand with your right side facing the wall, and extend your right arm overhead, palm flat against the wall.
- Take a tiny step back with your right foot and lean softly to the left.
- Concentrate on extending the right side of your torso and feeling a deep stretch along your latissimus dorsi muscle.
- To make the stretch as effective as possible, keep your chest open and your shoulders relaxed.
- Experiment with different angles and postures to get the best efficient stretch for your latissimus dorsi.
- Hold the stretch for 30 seconds to a minute, inhaling deeply and letting your muscles release any tension.
- Switch sides to stretch the left latissimus dorsi while maintaining symmetry and balance in your body.

Notes

Wall Neck Stretch

30 SECONDS.

Detailed Step by Step Instructions

- Stand facing the wall and press your right hand against it at shoulder level.
- Tilt your head to the left, bringing your left ear close to your left shoulder, until you feel a stretch on the right side of your neck.
- Instead of shrugging your shoulders or tensing your jaw, relax and stretch your neck muscles.
- Try gently pressing your hand against the wall to deepen the stretch, but only if it seems comfortable.
- Hold the stretch for 30 seconds while breathing deeply and evenly to encourage relaxation.
- Switch sides to stretch the right side of your neck while applying light yet steady pressure.
- Pay attention to any areas of tension or discomfort, and alter the stretch's intensity accordingly.

Notes

Wall Hamstring Stretch

2 MINUTES

Detailed Step by Step Instructions

- Lie on your back, hips near to the wall, legs extended upwards against the wall.
- Position your buttocks as near to the wall as possible while being comfortable.
- Maintain your legs straight and your feet flexed while feeling a slight stretch at the back of your thighs and calves.
- Experiment with altering the distance between your hips and the wall to find the best effective stretch for you.
- Hold the stretch for 1 to 2 minutes, focusing on relaxing your muscles and allowing the stretch to deepen gradually.
- Breathe deeply and evenly during the stretch, inhaling to expand your belly and expelling to relieve tension.
- If you're experiencing stiffness or tension in your lower back, consider placing a folded towel or cushion beneath your hips for support.

Notes

Wall Calf Stretch

30 SECONDS.

Detailed Step by Step Instructions

- Stand facing the wall, hands pushed on it at shoulder height for support.
- Step your right foot back about a foot from the wall and push your right heel into the ground.
- Keep your right leg straight and your foot level on the floor while leaning forward slightly, experiencing a stretch in your right calf.
- Experiment with changing the angle of your foot on the floor to target different parts of your calf muscle.
- Hold the stretch for 30 seconds, inhaling deeply until your muscles relax and extend.
- Switch sides to stretch the left leg while keeping symmetry and balance in your body.

Notes

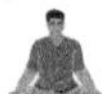

Wall Quadriceps Stretch

30 SECONDS.

Detailed Step by Step Instructions

- Stand facing away from the wall, feet hip-width apart, and hands pressed against the wall for support.
- Bend your right knee and reach back with your right hand to hold your right ankle.
- Gently draw your right heel towards your glutes until you feel a stretch in the front of your right leg.
- To ensure good alignment, keep your knees close together and your hips square to the wall.
- Experiment with altering the height of your foot against the wall to deepen the stretch as desired.
- Hold the stretch for 30 seconds, inhaling deeply until your muscles relax and extend.
- Switch sides to stretch the left quadriceps and ensure equal flexibility in both legs.

Notes

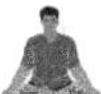

Wall Hip Flexor Stretch

30 SECONDS.

Detailed Step by Step Instructions

- Kneel on the ground, facing the wall, right knee against the wall, left foot flat on the floor in front of you.
- Place your hands on your hips to help your pelvis stay stable and in perfect position.
- Gently lean forward, maintaining your body upright and your pelvis neutral, until you feel a stretch at the front of your right hip.
- Avoid arching your lower back or sinking into your hips; instead, stretch the front of your hip flexors.
- Hold the stretch for 30 seconds, inhaling deeply and letting your muscles release any tension.
- Switch sides to stretch the left hip flexor while keeping symmetry and balance in your body.

Notes

Wall Triceps Stretch

30 SECONDS.

Detailed Step by Step Instructions

- Stand facing the wall, feet hip-width apart, arms stretched aloft.
- Bend your right elbow and extend your right hand down your back, flat on the wall.
- Gently press your right palm onto the wall while leaning to the left, feeling a stretch on the underside of your right arm.
- Keep your shoulders relaxed and your spine neutral, and prevent excessive twisting or arching.
- Experiment with varying the height of your arm on the wall to target different parts of your tricep.
- Hold the stretch for 30 seconds, inhaling deeply until your muscles relax and extend.
- Switch sides to stretch the left triceps while maintaining symmetry and balance in your body.

Notes

CHAPTER 5: CORE STRENGTHENING

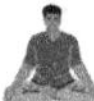

Core strength is essential for maintaining stability, balance, and appropriate posture throughout our daily lives. Wall Pilates exercises are an efficient technique to strengthen the core muscles while taking use of the support and resistance provided by the wall. These exercises work the muscles in the abdomen, lower back, hips, and pelvis, improving strength, endurance, and general functional movement.

Furthermore, strong core muscles are not only beneficial for physical health but also play a crucial role in preventing injuries, particularly in seniors. By strengthening the core, individuals can better support their spine and maintain stability during everyday activities, reducing the risk of falls and other accidents. Additionally, a strong core can contribute to better posture and alignment, which can alleviate back pain and improve overall quality of life.

Incorporating core-strengthening exercises into your routine can also enhance athletic performance and functional movement patterns. Whether you're an avid athlete or simply looking to stay active and independent as you age, a strong core is essential for performing activities such as walking, lifting, bending, and reaching with greater ease and efficiency. With consistent practice of Wall Pilates core exercises, you can build a solid foundation of strength and stability to support your active lifestyle and pursue your fitness goals with confidence.

In this chapter, we will look at twelve Wall Pilates exercises, each with thorough step-by-step instructions to ensure good form and maximum efficiency.

Wall Plank

30 SECONDS –1 MINUTE

Detailed Step by Step Instructions

- Begin by facing the wall, approximately an arm's length away.
- Place your hands on the wall at shoulder height and shoulder wide apart.
- Walk your feet back until your body forms a diagonal line from head to heels, then engage your core muscles.
- Press your palms firmly on the wall for 30 seconds to 1 minute.
- Keep your abdominals engaged and your spine neutral throughout the workout.
- To increase the difficulty, elevate one leg at a time or move your knees closer to your chest while remaining in the plank position.

Notes

Wall Sit-Up

1O –12 REPS

Detailed Step by Step Instructions

- Sit on the floor with your back to the wall, knees bent, and feet flat on the floor.
- Engage your core muscles and slowly move your feet away from the wall.
- Lower your torso to the floor, maintaining your back against the wall, and perform a sit-up motion.
- When your torso is parallel to the ground, carefully return to the beginning position.
- Repeat 10-12 times, focusing on controlled movement and a full range of motion.
- To avoid strain, keep your neck relaxed and your chin slightly tucked when performing the exercise.

Notes

Wall Roll-Up

8-10 REPS

Detailed Step by Step Instructions

- Lie on your back with your legs extended vertically against the wall, creating a 90-degree angle with your hips and knees.
- Extend your arms overhead and press your palms to the floor.
- Engage your core muscles and slowly move your spine off the floor, extending your fingertips to your toes.
- Slowly lower your spine back to the floor, one vertebra at a time, until you reach the beginning position.
- Repeat 8-10 times, focusing on smooth, controlled movement and keeping your lower back in contact with the floor throughout the exercise.

Notes

Wall Side Plank

30 SECONDS –1 MINUTE

Detailed Step by Step Instructions

- Begin by standing sideways to the wall, left side facing it.
- Place your left forearm on the wall at shoulder level, elbow just beneath your shoulder.
- Step back and stack your feet on top of one another, balancing on the outside edge of your left foot.
- Lift your hips towards the ceiling, forming a straight line from head to heels.
- Hold this stance for 30 seconds to a minute, engaging your obliques while remaining stable.
- Repeat on the opposing side, taking equal time and effort on both sides of the body.

Notes

Wall Bicycle Crunch

10-12 REPS

Detailed Step by Step Instructions

- Lie on your back, hips near to the wall, legs extended vertically against it.
- Position your hands behind your head, elbows pointed to the sides.
- Engage your core muscles and lift your shoulders off the floor, bringing your right elbow to your left knee and straightening your right leg.
- While switching legs in a pedaling motion, rotate your torso to bring your left elbow nearer your right knee.
- Continue switching sides for 10-12 repetitions, keeping your core stable and moving with control.

Notes

Wall Pike

30 SECONDS –1 MINUTE

Detailed Step by Step Instructions

- Begin in a plank position with your feet against the wall and your hands on the floor shoulder-width apart.
- Engage your core muscles and push your hips to the ceiling while keeping your legs straight.
- To maintain stability, press through your palms and hold the inverted "V" position for 30 seconds to 1 minute.
- Lift your tailbone towards the sky and press your heels against the wall to increase the stretch in your hamstrings and calves.

Notes

Wall Mountain Climbers

30 SECONDS –1 MINUTE

Detailed Step by Step Instructions

- Begin in a plank stance facing the wall, hands shoulder-width apart and feet hip-width apart.
- Engage your core muscles and bring your right knee to your chest while keeping your back straight and hips level.
- Quickly switch legs, lowering your left knee to your chest and extending your right leg back to its original position.
- Continue alternating legs in a rapid, rhythmic motion for 30 seconds to 1 minute, keeping your core and shoulders stable.

Notes

Wall Russian Twist

10-12 REPS

Detailed Step by Step Instructions

- Sit on the floor with your back to the wall, knees bent, and feet flat on the floor.
- Lean back slightly to engage your core muscles, then lift your feet off the floor, balancing on your sit bones.
- Clasp your hands in front of your chest or use a weight to enhance resistance.
- Rotate your torso to the right, directing your clasped hands or weight toward the wall beside you.
- Return to the center, then turn to the left, bringing your hands or weight to the opposite wall.
- Continue switching sides for 10-12 repetitions, emphasizing controlled movement and balance.

Notes

Wall Leg Raise

10–12 REPS

Detailed Step by Step Instructions

- Lie on your back, hips near to the wall, legs extended vertically against it.
- Place your hands behind your hips for support, palms down.
- Engage your core muscles and pull your legs straight up towards the ceiling.
- Slowly lower your legs back to the wall, pausing a few inches above the floor.
- Lift your legs back up towards the ceiling, keeping your core stable and moving with control.
- Repeat 10-12 times, keeping your lower back pressed against the floor during the exercise.

Notes

Wall Lunge Twist

10 –12 REPS

Detailed Step by Step Instructions

- Stand facing away from the wall, feet hip-width apart, and hands clasped in front of your chest.
- Take a large step forward with your right foot, then lower into a lunge position, bending both knees to 90 degrees.
- Press your palms together and rotate your torso to the right, bringing your clasped hands to the wall next to you.
- Return to the center, then spin to the left, bringing your hands to the opposite wall.
- Continue alternating sides for 10-12 reps, keeping your core stable and your chest raised.

Notes

Wall Knee Tuck

10 –12 REPS

Detailed Step by Step Instructions

- Begin in a plank stance facing the wall, hands shoulder-width apart and feet hip-width apart.
- Engage your core muscles and bring your right knee up to your chest, slightly curving your spine.
- Hold this stance for a time before extending your right leg back to its initial position.
- Repeat with your left knee, pulling it towards your chest before stretching it back.
- Continue alternating legs for 10-12 repetitions, keeping your core and shoulders stable.

Notes

Wall Bridge

30 SECONDS –1 MINUTE

Detailed Step by Step Instructions

- Lie on your back, feet flat on the floor, knees bent, hip-width apart.
- Place your arms by your sides, palms pressed into the floor.
- Lift your hips towards the ceiling while engaging your core muscles, forming a straight line from your shoulders to your knees.
- Press through your heels to activate your glutes and hamstrings, then hold this bridge position for 30 seconds to 1 minute.
- Maintain a neutral spine and prevent overarching or tilting the pelvis.
- To increase the intensity, elevate one leg at a time or place a tiny weight on your hips.

Notes

CHAPTER 6: UPPER BODY STRENGTH

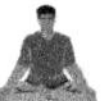

Upper body strength is necessary for performing daily tasks, keeping excellent posture, and improving athletic performance. Wall exercises are a handy and effective technique to target upper-body muscles such as the chest, shoulders, back, and arms while utilizing minimal equipment. Using the resistance produced by a wall allows you to efficiently challenge and build your muscles while increasing stability and coordination. Moreover, enhancing upper body strength through wall exercises can have significant benefits for individuals of all ages, particularly seniors. As we age, maintaining muscle mass and strength becomes increasingly important for preserving independence and quality of life. Strong upper body muscles can make daily tasks such as lifting groceries, carrying grandchildren, or even getting up from a chair much easier and safer. By incorporating targeted wall exercises into your routine, you can build and maintain the strength needed to stay active and independent as you age.

In addition to functional benefits, improving upper body strength can also have a positive impact on overall health and well-being. Research has shown that individuals with greater muscle strength tend to have lower rates of chronic diseases such as heart disease, diabetes, and osteoporosis. By engaging in regular upper body wall workouts, you not only strengthen your muscles but also support your long-term health and vitality. Plus, the sense of accomplishment and empowerment that comes with mastering new exercises and seeing improvements in strength can boost confidence and enhance overall quality of life.

In this chapter, we'll look at twelve upper body wall workouts, each with precise step-by-step instructions to ensure good form and maximum efficiency.

Wall Push-Up

10-12 REPS

Detailed Step by Step Instructions

- Begin by facing the wall at arm's length, feet hip-width apart.
- Position your hands on the wall at shoulder height, somewhat wider than shoulder width apart.
- Engage your core muscles and take a step back, making a little angle with the wall.
- Bend your elbows and lower your chest towards the wall while keeping them close to your sides.
- Straighten your arms by pressing through your palms, then return to the beginning posture.
- Repeat 10-12 times, focusing on controlled movement and keeping a straight line from head to heels.

Notes

Wall Handstand Hold

30 SECONDS –1 MINUTE

Detailed Step by Step Instructions

- Face away from the wall, with your feet hip-width apart and your hands on the floor shoulder-width apart.
- Walk your feet up the wall until your body forms an inverted "V" configuration, with your hips piled over your shoulders.
- Lift your shoulders off the floor by pressing with your palms and fingertips, utilizing your core muscles.
- Maintain this handstand position for 30 seconds to 1 minute, focusing on stability and alignment.
- To enhance the intensity, try pulling one knee to your chest or elevating one leg towards the ceiling while retaining the handstand position.

Notes

Wall Shoulder Press

10–12 REPS

Detailed Step by Step Instructions

- Stand facing the wall, feet hip-width apart, arms extended aloft, palms facing forward.
- Press your palms against the wall and steadily lower your body towards it while bending your elbows.
- As you lower your body, keep your core engaged and your spine neutral. You should feel a stretch in your shoulders and chest.
- Straighten your arms by pressing through your palms, then return to the beginning posture.
- Repeat 10-12 times, focusing on controlled movement and keeping tension in your shoulder muscles.

Notes

Wall Pike Push-Up

10-12 REPS

Detailed Step by Step Instructions

- Begin in a plank stance facing the wall, hands shoulder-width apart and feet hip-width apart.
- Walk your feet toward the wall until your body forms an inverted "V" shape, with your hips raised to the ceiling.
- Bend your elbows and lower your head to the floor while maintaining a straight line.
- Straighten your arms by pressing through your palms, then return to the beginning posture.
- Repeat 10-12 times, paying special attention to controlled movement and core and shoulder stability.

Notes

Wall Chest Press

10-12 REPS

Detailed Step by Step Instructions

- Stand facing away from the wall, with your feet hip-width apart and your hands at shoulder height against the wall.
- Lean slightly forward and bend your elbows, bringing your chest to the wall.
- Straighten your arms and push yourself away from the wall by pressing through your hands.
- Repeat 10-12 times, focusing on controlled movement and keeping tension in your chest muscles.

Notes

Wall Triceps Dip

10–12 REPS

Detailed Step by Step Instructions

- Sit on the floor with your back to the wall, knees bent, and feet flat on the floor.
- Place your hands on the wall behind you, shoulder height, fingers pointing toward your body.
- Lift your hips off the floor and walk your feet forward, forming a tiny angle between your body and the wall.
- Bend your elbows and lower yourself toward the wall, experiencing a stretch in your triceps.
- Straighten your arms by pressing through your palms, then return to the beginning posture.
- Repeat 10-12 times, paying special attention to controlled movement and core and shoulder stability.

Notes

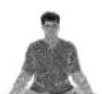

Wall Pull-Up

8-10 REPS

Detailed Step by Step Instructions

- Stand facing the wall, feet hip-width apart, arms extended aloft, palms facing forward.
- Reach up and grasp the top of the wall with an overhand grip, keeping your hands slightly wider than shoulder width apart.
- Pull your chest towards the wall, bending your elbows and lifting your chin over the wall's level.
- Lower yourself back down with control until your arms are completely extended.
- Repeat 8-10 times, focusing on controlled movement and keeping tension in your back and arms.

Notes

Wall Bicep Curl

10-12 REPS

Detailed Step by Step Instructions

- Stand facing the wall, feet hip-width apart, arms extended aloft, palms facing forward.
- Position your hands on the wall at shoulder height, somewhat wider than shoulder width apart.
- Bend your elbows and curl your hands towards your shoulders while keeping your upper arms motionless against the wall.
- Lower your hands back down carefully until your arms are fully stretched.
- Repeat 10-12 times, focusing on controlled movement and keeping your biceps tight.

Notes

Wall Shoulder Stretch

30 SECONDS –1 MINUTE

Detailed Step by Step Instructions

- Stand sideways to the wall, right side facing it.
- Extend your right arm and rest your palm flat against the wall, shoulder height.
- Slowly twist your body away from the wall while maintaining your arm extended until you feel a stretch in your shoulders and chest.
- Hold for 30 seconds to one minute, then switch sides.

Notes

Wall Lateral Raise

10-12 REPS

Detailed Step by Step Instructions

- Stand facing the wall, feet hip-width apart, arms extended aloft, palms facing forward.
- Position your hands on the wall at shoulder height, somewhat wider than shoulder width apart.
- Engage your core muscles and raise your arms to the sides until they are parallel to the ground.
- Lower your arms back down with control until completely extended.
- Repeat 10-12 times, concentrating on controlled movement and maintaining tension in your shoulders.

Notes

Wall Pike Hold

10 REPS

Detailed Step by Step Instructions

- Begin in a plank stance facing the wall, hands shoulder-width apart and feet hip-width apart.
- Walk your feet toward the wall until your body forms an inverted "V" shape, with your hips raised to the ceiling.
- Lift your shoulders off the floor by pressing with your palms and fingertips, utilizing your core muscles.
- Maintain this pike position for 30 seconds to 1 minute, focusing on stability and alignment.

Notes

Wall Chest Fly

10–12 REPS

Detailed Step by Step Instructions

- Stand facing the wall, feet hip-width apart, arms extended aloft, palms facing forward.
- Reach out and grab the sides of the wall with an overhand grip, keeping your hands slightly wider than shoulder width apart.
- Pull your chest towards the wall while engaging your core muscles. Bring your hands together in front of you.
- Slowly release and return to the beginning posture, keeping tension in your chest muscles.
- Repeat 10-12 times, paying special attention to controlled movement and core and shoulder stability.

Notes

CHAPTER 7: LOWER BODY STRENGTH

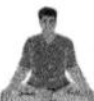

Stability, mobility, and general functional movement all require lower-body strength development. Wall exercises are a unique and effective approach to target the muscles of the legs, hips, and glutes while just using a wall for support and resistance. These workouts may be performed anywhere with minimum room and equipment, making them suitable for people of all fitness levels.

Furthermore, building lower body strength through wall exercises is particularly beneficial for improving balance and reducing the risk of falls, especially among seniors. As we age, maintaining strong and stable legs becomes essential for staying mobile and independent. Strengthening the muscles of the legs, hips, and glutes can help support proper alignment and stability, allowing individuals to navigate uneven terrain, stairs, and other obstacles with greater ease and confidence. By incorporating targeted lower body wall exercises into your routine, you can enhance your balance and mobility, reducing the likelihood of accidents and injuries.

Additionally, developing lower body strength can enhance performance in various sports and physical activities, from hiking and cycling to dancing and gardening. Strong legs and glutes provide a solid foundation for dynamic movements and explosive power, allowing athletes and active individuals to excel in their chosen pursuits. Whether you're a weekend warrior or simply looking to stay active and mobile as you age, strengthening the lower body through wall exercises can help you move more efficiently, improve endurance, and enjoy a higher quality of life.

In this chapter, we will look at eleven lower body wall exercises, each with precise step-by-step instructions to ensure good form and maximum efficiency.

Wall Sit

30 SECONDS –1 MINUTE

Detailed Step by Step Instructions

- Start by standing with your back to the wall and your feet hip-width apart.
- Lower your body to a seated position, sliding your back down the wall until your thighs are parallel to the ground.
- Maintain a neutral spine and knee-ankle alignment, avoiding back rounding or arching.
- Maintain this seated position for 30 seconds to 1 minute, concentrating on activating your quadriceps, hamstrings, and glutes.
- Press through your heels to return to the beginning posture, and repeat for several sets.

Notes

Wall Calf Raise

10-12 REPS

Detailed Step by Step Instructions

- Stand facing the wall, your feet hip-width apart, and your hands rest lightly against the wall for support.
- Lift your heels off the floor and as far up onto the balls of your feet as you can.
- Hold this lifted stance for a moment, then descend your heels back to the floor.
- Repeat 10-12 times, focusing on controlled movement and maintaining ankle and calves stability.

Notes

Wall Hamstring Curl

10–12 REPS

Detailed Step by Step Instructions

- Lie on your back, hips near to the wall, feet flat against it, knees bent.
- For support, press your palms into the floor and lift your hips off the floor, forming a straight line from shoulders to knees.
- Engage your core muscles and steadily glide your feet down the wall until your legs are fully stretched.
- Bend your knees and bend your heels toward your glutes, then slide your feet back up the wall.
- Repeat 10-12 times, paying special attention to controlled movement and core and hip stability.

Notes

Wall Lunge

10–12 REPS

Detailed Step by Step Instructions

- Stand facing the wall, your feet hip-width apart, and your hands rest lightly against the wall for support.
- Take a large step back with your right foot, then drop your body into a lunge position, bending both knees to 90 degrees.
- Keep your front knee in line with your ankle and your back knee hanging slightly above the floor.
- Return to the beginning posture by pressing through your front heel.
- Repeat 10-12 times on each leg, alternating sides.

Notes

Wall Single Leg Bridge

10-12 REPS

Detailed Step by Step Instructions

- Lie on your back, hips near to the wall, knees bent, and feet flat on the floor.
- Extend your right leg straight up to the ceiling, placing the sole of your foot into the wall.
- Lift your hips towards the ceiling by pressing your left foot, forming a straight line from shoulders to knees.
- Hold this bridge position for a moment, then descend your hips back to the floor.
- Repeat 10-12 times on each leg, alternating sides.

Notes

Wall Side Lunge

10–12 REPS

Detailed Step by Step Instructions

- Stand sideways to the wall, right side facing it, and feet wider than hip width apart.
- Place your right hand against the wall for support, then take a large stride to the left, bending your left knee and lowering your body into a side lunge.
- Keep your left knee in line with your ankle and your right leg straight.
- Stand back up to the beginning position by pressing through your left heel.
- Repeat 10-12 times on each leg, alternating sides.

Notes

Wall Leg Press

10-12 REPS

Detailed Step by Step Instructions

- Lie on your back, hips near to the wall, knees bent, and feet flat on the floor.
- Extend your right leg straight up to the ceiling, placing the sole of your foot into the wall.
- Lift your hips towards the ceiling by pressing your left foot, forming a straight line from shoulders to knees.
- Hold this bridge position for a moment, then descend your hips back to the floor.
- Repeat 10-12 times on each leg, alternating sides.

Notes

Wall Bulgarian Split Squat

10–12 REPS

Detailed Step by Step Instructions

- Stand facing away from the wall, with your right foot against the wall behind you and your left foot firmly planted on the ground in front of you.
- Lower your body into a split squat, bending your left knee to 90 degrees and maintaining your right knee slightly above the floor.
- Stand back up to the beginning position by pressing through your left heel.
- Repeat 10-12 times on each leg, alternating sides.

Notes

Wall Sumo Squat

10–12 REPS

Detailed Step by Step Instructions

- Stand facing the wall, feet wider than hip-width apart, toes turned out at a 45-degree angle.
- Place your hands on the wall for support and lower yourself into a sumo squat position, bending your knees and lowering your hips to the floor.
- Keep your chest high and your spine neutral, with no rounding or arching of the back.
- Stand back up to the beginning position by pressing through your heels.
- Repeat 10-12 times, focusing on controlled movement and keeping tension in your inner thighs and glutes.

Notes

Wall Glute Bridge

30 SECONDS –1 MINUTE

Detailed Step by Step Instructions

- Lie on your back, hips near to the wall, knees bent, and feet flat on the floor.
- Place your arms by your sides, palms pressed into the floor.
- Create a straight line from shoulders to knees by engaging your core muscles and lifting your hips toward the ceiling.
- Press through your heels to activate your glutes and hamstrings, then hold this bridge position for 30 seconds to 1 minute.
- Maintain a neutral spine and prevent overarching or tilting the pelvis.

Notes

Wall Pistol Squat

10-12 REPS

Detailed Step by Step Instructions

- Stand facing away from the wall, feet hip-width apart, arms extended straight out in front of you.
- Lift your right leg off the floor and extend it straight out in front of you, parallel to the ground.
- Lower your body into a squat position with your left leg, bending your left knee and lowering your hips to the floor.
- Stand back up to the beginning position by pressing through your left heel.
- Repeat 10-12 times on each leg, alternating sides.

Notes

CHAPTER 8: BALANCE AND STABILITY

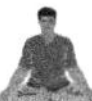

Balance and stability are critical components of total fitness, allowing you to complete daily activities and avoid accidents. Wall exercises create a supportive environment for improving balance and stability by using the wall for aid and feedback. These exercises work the muscles in the core, legs, and hips while testing proprioception and coordination.

Moreover, improving balance and stability through wall exercises is especially beneficial for older adults who may experience declines in these areas due to aging or certain medical conditions. As we age, maintaining good balance becomes increasingly important for preventing falls and maintaining independence. By regularly practicing balance-enhancing wall exercises, seniors can strengthen the muscles involved in stability and refine their proprioceptive skills, reducing the risk of falls and enhancing confidence in everyday activities.

In addition to physical benefits, enhancing balance and stability can also have a positive impact on mental well-being. Research has shown that individuals with better balance tend to experience greater feelings of confidence, independence, and overall quality of life. By incorporating balance-improving wall exercises into your routine, you not only support your physical health but also boost your mental resilience and sense of empowerment. Plus, the mindfulness and concentration required to perform these exercises can promote relaxation and stress relief, helping you feel more centered and grounded in your daily life.

In this chapter, we'll look at nine wall exercises that improve balance and stability, each with precise step-by-step instructions to ensure appropriate technique and maximum efficiency.

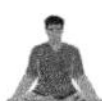

Wall Single Leg Balance

30 SECONDS –1 MINUTE

Detailed Step by Step Instructions

- Stand facing the wall, your feet hip-width apart, and your hands rest lightly against the wall for support.
- Lift your right foot off the floor while balancing on your left leg.
- Engage your core muscles and keep a straight line from head to heel, with no bending or tilting.
- Maintain this single-leg balance for 30 seconds to a minute, concentrating on stability and control.
- Switch over and perform the exercise with your right leg.

Notes

Wall Plank with Leg Lift

10-12 REPS

Detailed Step by Step Instructions

- Begin in a plank stance facing the wall, hands shoulder-width apart and feet hip-width apart.
- Engage your core muscles and raise your right leg off the ground, stretching it straight behind you.
- Hold this single-leg plank for a moment before lowering your right leg back to the floor.
- Repeat the leg lift 10-12 times on your right leg, focusing on stability and control.
- Switch over and perform the exercise with your left leg.

Notes

Wall Knee Drives

10–12 REPS

Detailed Step by Step Instructions

- Stand facing the wall, your feet hip-width apart, and your hands rest lightly against the wall for support.
- Lift your right knee to your chest, driving it towards the wall, and then return to the starting position.
- Repeat the knee drives for 10-12 times on your right leg, focusing on controlled movement and balance.
- Switch over and perform the exercise with your left leg.

Notes

Wall Side Leg Raise

10–12 REPS

Detailed Step by Step Instructions

- Stand sideways to the wall, right side facing it, feet together.
- Place your right hand against the wall for support and lift your left leg out to the side while keeping it straight.
- Hold the side leg raise for a second before lowering your left leg back to the starting position.
- Repeat the leg lift 10-12 times on your left leg, focusing on stability and control.
- Switch over and perform the exercise with your right leg.

Notes

10–12 REPS

Detailed Step by Step Instructions

- Stand sideways to the wall, right side facing it, feet together.
- Swing your left leg out to the side, then back across your torso, while supporting yourself with your right hand against the wall.
- Repeat the leg swing 10-12 times on your left leg, focusing on controlled movement and balance.
- Switch over and perform the exercise with your right leg.

Notes

Wall Stability Ball Hold

30 SECONDS –1 MINUTE

Detailed Step by Step Instructions

- Stand facing the wall, your feet hip-width apart, and your hands rest lightly against the wall for support.
- Place a stability ball between your lower back and the wall, then press into it.
- Engage your core muscles and grip this stability ball for 30 seconds to 1 minute, concentrating on stability and control.

Notes

Wall Mountain Pose

30 SECONDS –1 MINUTE

Detailed Step by Step Instructions

- Stand facing the wall, your feet hip-width apart, and your hands rest lightly against the wall for support.
- Press your palms against the wall and walk your feet back until your body forms an inverted "V" shape.
- Hold this mountain posture for 30 seconds to a minute, concentrating on stability and balance.

Notes

Wall Hip Abduction

10-12 REPS

Detailed Step by Step Instructions

- Stand facing the wall, your feet hip-width apart, and your hands rest lightly against the wall for support.
- Lift your right leg to the side while keeping it straight, then return to the starting position.
- Repeat the hip abduction on your right leg 10-12 times, focusing on controlled movement and balance.
- Switch over and perform the exercise with your left leg.

Notes

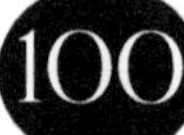

Wall Hip Extension

10–12 REPS

Detailed Step by Step Instructions

- Stand facing the wall, your feet hip-width apart, and your hands rest lightly against the wall for support.
- Lift your right leg straight back behind you, squeezing your glutes at the top, and then return to the beginning position.
- Repeat the hip extension 10-12 times on your right leg, focusing on controlled movement and balance.
- Switch over and perform the exercise with your left leg.

Notes

CHAPTER 9: COOL DOWN AND STRETCH

incorporating a thorough cool-down and stretching routine is essential for promoting muscle recovery, reducing discomfort, and enhancing flexibility and range of motion. Wall exercises offer a practical and effective way to stretch and relax your muscles, leveraging the support and feedback provided by a wall.

During a cool-down session, the body transitions from a state of heightened activity to a more relaxed state. This gradual reduction in intensity allows the heart rate and breathing rate to return to normal levels, while also aiding in the removal of metabolic waste products from the muscles. Additionally, stretching during the cool-down helps to alleviate muscle tension and soreness, preventing stiffness and promoting faster recovery.

Wall exercises provide a unique opportunity to incorporate both static and dynamic stretching techniques into your cool-down routine. By using the wall as a prop, you can safely and effectively target specific muscle groups, allowing for a deeper and more controlled stretch. Whether you're focusing on the hamstrings, quadriceps, calves, or shoulders, the wall can provide support and stability as you move through various stretching exercises.

Furthermore, wall exercises can help improve proprioception and body awareness, allowing you to better understand and control your range of motion. By gently pressing into the wall or using it to guide your movements, you can enhance your sense of spatial orientation and alignment, leading to safer and more effective stretching.

In this chapter, we'll explore a comprehensive cool-down and stretching routine using wall exercises.

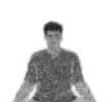

Wall Forward Fold

30 SECONDS –1 MINUTE

Detailed Step by Step Instructions

- Stand facing the wall, your feet hip-width apart.
- Place your palms flat against the wall, shoulder height.
- Walk your hands down the wall, lean forward at the hips, and keep your back straight.
- Continue to walk your hands down the wall until you feel a stretch at the back of your legs and spine.
- Hold this stretch for 30 seconds to a minute, focusing on relaxing into it and breathing deeply.

Notes

Wall Butterfly Stretch

30 SECONDS –1 MINUTE

Detailed Step by Step Instructions

- Sit on the floor, facing the wall, knees bent and soles of your feet together.
- Press the bottoms of your feet on the wall and slide your heels closer to your torso.
- Gently press your knees down to the floor, experiencing a stretch in your inner thighs and groin.
- Hold this stretch for 30 seconds to a minute, focusing on relaxing and breathing deeply.

Notes

Wall Figure Four Stretch

30 SECONDS –1 MINUTE

Detailed Step by Step Instructions

- Lie on your back, hips close to the wall, knees bent.
- Place your right ankle on top of your left knee to form a "figure four" formation with your legs.
- Slide your left foot down the wall, feeling a stretch in your right hip and glutes.
- Hold this stretch for 30 seconds to a minute before switching sides and repeating on the left side.

Notes

Wall Spinal Twist

30 SECONDS –1 MINUTE

Detailed Step by Step Instructions

- Sit on the floor, facing the wall, with your legs extended straight in front of you.
- Bend your right knee and cross your right foot across your left leg, keeping it flat on the floor.
- Twist your torso to the right, placing your left elbow on the outside of your right knee.
- Press your elbow into your knee as you twist your upper body to the right, experiencing a stretch down your spine and outer hip.
- Hold this stretch for 30 seconds to 1 minute before switching sides and repeating on the left side.

Notes

Wall Child's Pose

30 SECONDS –1 MINUTE

Detailed Step by Step Instructions

- Kneel on the floor, toes together and knees hip-width apart, facing the wall.
- Sit back on your heels and reach your arms forward, palms flat against the wall at shoulder level.
- Lower your forehead to the ground and relax your chest toward your thighs, experiencing a stretch in your back and shoulders.
- Hold this stretch for 30 seconds to 1 minute, concentrating on deepening your breathing and relaxing into the position.

Notes

CHAPTER 10: CONCLUSION AND TIPS FOR CONTINUED PRACTICE

Congratulations on successfully completing your Wall Pilates experience! In this last chapter, we'll look back on your accomplishments, go over the basic principles of Wall Pilates, and offer advice on how to maintain and grow your practice in the next days, weeks, and months.

Throughout this guide, you've studied the essential principles of Wall Pilates as well as a range of exercises and strategies for strengthening your body, increasing flexibility, and improving your general well-being. From the significance of posture to the advantages of using the wall as a prop, you've learned vital insights and practical techniques to help you with your Pilates practice.

As you continue your Pilates journey beyond this book, here are some pointers to keep you inspired, interested, and devoted to the practice:

Set Realistic Goals: Define specific and attainable goals for your Pilates practice, such as improving posture, increasing flexibility, or developing core strength. Break down your goals into smaller, more doable steps and celebrate your accomplishments along the way.

Prioritize Consistency: Make Pilates a regular part of your routine by setting aside time for practice each day or week. Consistency is essential for achieving outcomes, so commit to showing up for yourself and your health.

Listen to your body. Pay attention to how your body feels during your Pilates session and alter your regimen accordingly. If something does not feel right or causes discomfort, change the activity or take a break. Respect your body's requirements and limitations.

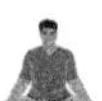

Stay Curious and Open-Minded: Approach your Pilates practice with curiosity and openness, trying out new exercises, variations, and techniques. Accept obstacles as opportunities for growth and discovery, and do not be scared to leave your comfort zone.

Seek Support and direction: Consider working with a certified Pilates instructor or enrolling in a Pilates class to obtain personalized direction, feedback, and support. A knowledgeable instructor can help you improve your technique, answer any questions or concerns, and keep you motivated and accountable.

Incorporate Mindfulness: Use your Pilates practice to promote mindfulness and present by paying attention to the sensations in your body and the rhythm of your breathing. Mindful movement can help you connect with your body and have a deeper understanding of Pilates.

Mix it up: Experiment with different styles, equipment, and environments to keep your Pilates practice interesting and fresh. Experiment with mat Pilates, equipment-based Pilates, and other mind-body modalities to find what works for you.

Celebrate Your Progress: Take time to recognize and celebrate your accomplishments, no matter how minor. Whether you're mastering a difficult exercise, expanding your flexibility, or simply committing to regular practice, every step forward is worth celebrating.

Stay Inspired: Surround yourself with sources of inspiration to help you stay motivated and involved in your Pilates practice. Discover what inspires and fuels your passion for movement, whether it's by reading books, watching videos, attending seminars, or interacting with other Pilates fans.

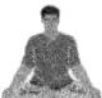

Enjoy the journey: Above all, remember to enjoy the Pilates journey—the process of learning, growing, and expanding in both body and mind. Approach your practice with joy, gratitude, and curiosity, and allow it to transform your life in unexpected ways.

As you continue to practice Pilates beyond this guide, keep in mind that the advantages go far beyond the physical realm. Pilates is a comprehensive discipline that benefits the mind, body, and soul, building a stronger connection with yourself and the world around you. Accept each minute on the mat as a time for self-discovery, self-care, and self-improvement, and allow your Pilates practice to bring you strength, vitality, and joy in your life.

Thank you for joining us on this trip, and best wishes for continued success and fulfillment on your Pilates route. May your practice motivate, encourage, and empower you to live your best life, and may your journey be filled with health, pleasure, and abundance.

Namaste,
Jerry Hargrave

A GIFT TO OUR READERS

As a symbol of our appreciation for joining us on this path to better health and vitality, we'd like to give you a unique gift: a free 4-week planner to help you track your progress and keep organized during your Wall Pilates workout.

This planner is your personal success tool, allowing you to organize your workouts, establish realistic objectives, and monitor your progress over the next four weeks. This planner, with specific area to record your workouts, maintain your measurements, and jot down any notes or observations, will be your buddy along the journey.

We believe that consistency and responsibility are essential for reaching your fitness objectives, and this calendar is meant to help you every step of the way. Whether you're just starting out with Wall Pilates or want to take your practice to the next level, this schedule will keep you focused, motivated, and on track to achieve your goals

Jerry Hargrave,
CompanionLit Wellness Team

WEEK 1   Wall Pilates Fitness Planner

DAY	EXERCISE	GOAL
Monday		
Tuesday		
Wednesday		
Thursday		
Friday		
Saturday		
Sunday		

 Wall Pilates Fitness Planner

DAY	EXERCISE	GOAL
Monday		
Tuesday		
Wednesday		
Thursday		
Friday		
Saturday		
Sunday		

WEEK 3   Wall Pilates Fitness Planner

DAY	EXERCISE	GOAL
Monday		
Tuesday		
Wednesday		
Thursday		
Friday		
Saturday		
Sunday		

 Wall Pilates Fitness Planner

DAY	EXERCISE	GOAL
Monday		
Tuesday		
Wednesday		
Thursday		
Friday		
Saturday		
Sunday		

www.ingramcontent.com/pod-product-compliance
Lightning Source LLC
Chambersburg PA
CBHW081550250726
48653CB00009B/3356